Praise for *Gone Before Gone*

"Jerri Clark writes beautifully, with solid information and enlightening stories. She teaches in a way that is clear and conceptually correct. Whether readers are facing SMI or other unresolvable ambiguous losses, they will be empowered by this book."
> — Pauline Boss, PhD, author of *Ambiguous Loss*;
> *Loss, Trauma, and Resilience*; and *The Myth of Closure*

"Jerri Clark has written an important book. What is most unusual is her detailed account of coming to grips with her loss, as she "stopped begging the universe to reverse time and give me my old life back." I have read books on schizophrenia and bipolar disorder for over fifty years and would rank this book in the top five percent for families."
> — E. Fuller Torrey, MD, author of *American Psychosis*,
> *Surviving Schizophrenia*, and *Surviving Manic Depression*

"*Gone Before Gone* is an extraordinary and searching book that combines Jerri Clark's narrative of struggle and loss with acute glimpses into the chaotic universe of mental healthcare in America. Families with stricken children on the precipice of this murky, confounding universe will find themselves guided toward healing with intelligence and warmth."
> — Ron Powers, author of *No One Cares About Crazy People*

"This book will reach a wide swath of readers, who will come away with empathy and insight into those who live with mental illness, along with their families. Jerri Clark has lived, and survived, every parent's worst nightmare. This book powerfully and poignantly delineates how to navigate through and beyond ambiguous loss."
> — Gail Freedman, producer of the movie
> *No One Cares About Crazy People*

"This book should be read by everyone who encounters people with mental illness in their work. We have built the largest psychiatry training program in the U.S. here at UW: I want all of our residents to read this book at the beginning of their careers."

— Jürgen Unützer, MD, chair of psychiatry
at the University of Washington

"A powerful and deeply compassionate read, *Gone Before Gone* gives voice to what so many families live but struggle to name: the quiet grief of loving and missing someone who is still here yet changed by severe mental illness."

— Ann Corcoran, RN, MSN, Executive Director,
National Shattering Silence Coalition

"Jerri Clark writes with rare honesty, weaving grief, love, and hard-won insight into a narrative that both breaks and strengthens the reader's heart. This book belongs on everyone's bookshelf because it cultivates empathy, understanding, and the kind of courage we all need."

— Nicole Drapeau Gillen, author of *Schizophrenia and*
Other Related Disorders: A Handbook for Caregivers

"What Jerri Clark has written is horrifically beautiful. It heartachingly tells what so many of us have been trying to express. An army of moms (and other family members) need this book."

— Sherri Wittwer, Utah family advocate

"*Gone Before Gone* is deeply personal, painfully honest, and incredibly useful. Jerri writes with fierce clarity and hard-won compassion, giving families living with SMI the tools they've been denied for far too long. This is essential reading."

— Todd Brown, award-winning author of
When Shadows Burn

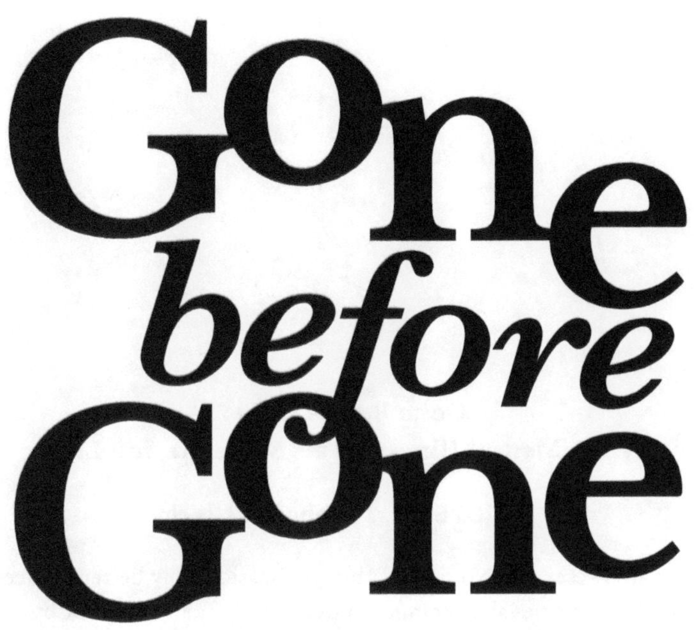

Gone before Gone

When Mental Illness Steals Someone You Love

Jerri Niebaum Clark

Gone before Gone

When Mental Illness Steals Someone You Love

Jerri Niebaum Clark

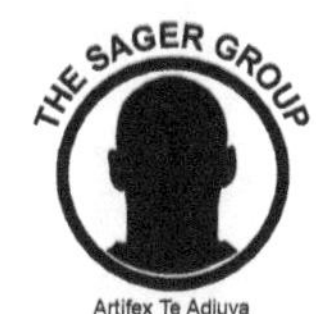

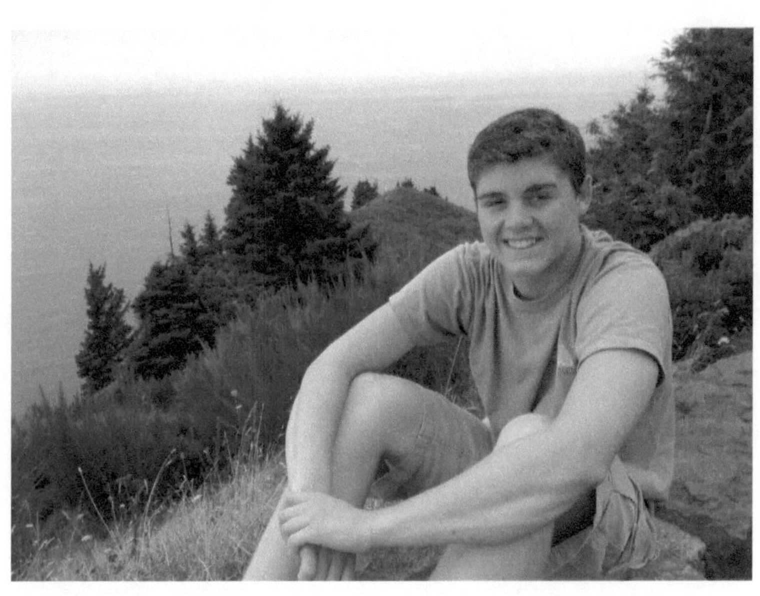

This book is dedicated to my son, Calvin Clark.
He was born November 28, 1995, and died March 18, 2019.

Author's Note

Pauline Boss, PhD, professor emeritus of family social science at the University of Minnesota and a long-time family therapist, coined the term "ambiguous loss" and introduced core theories and concepts referenced in this book. The six coping guidelines are labeled with phrases that are of Boss' invention: "make meaning," "adjust mastery," "reconstruct identity," "revise attachment," "normalize ambivalence," and "find new hope."

Dr. Boss developed the concept of "both, and..." thinking. I also learned from her that a person might be "gone but not gone." From her I learned to apply these terms: "let go while remembering," "absolute identity," "idealized relationships," and "what is real may not be ideal." I also learned to consider how one might "play with ambiguity" and "discover what is still possible, despite not getting what was originally wanted."

After learning these and other core concepts from Dr. Boss, I applied the terminology for myself and other families like mine who live with unimaginable losses caused by complex mental illness circumstances within our families. As a non-clinician, I adapted the terms in ways that felt family friendly and practical and often used them in combination with self-help techniques learned elsewhere or through personal exploration.

When it comes to ambiguous loss, Dr. Boss is the unrivaled expert. I am unapologetically her acolyte, a disciple of her principles and a devoted fan. I'm honored to have learned directly from her by completing her certification course, offered by the University of Minnesota's Department of Family Social Science. This nomenclature has enabled me to give structure to my own coping and to better guide others through seminars I offer as part of my job as a resource and advocacy manager at Treatment Advocacy Center (TAC).

Ambiguousloss.com is a website built by Dr. Boss and maintained by the University of Minnesota's Department of Family Social Science. That website is a good place to learn more about books by Dr. Boss, many of which are also listed in the appendices of this book. Thank you, Dr. Boss, for offering a method for healing with ambiguous loss.

Foreword

Jerri Niebaum Clark loved her son, Calvin, from the moment he was born. She changed his diapers, sang him to sleep at night, and felt the pure joy that came when he first said "Mommy." When Calvin later described his childhood, he pictured "a smiling sun in a cutely drawn neighborhood—everything a kid would ever want." There were good schools, plenty of friends, and endless smiles. Jerri taught Calvin how to surf—one of her passions—and watched with pride as he caught his first wave. Family vacations and birthdays were joyful celebrations. There were hiccups, of course—the ordinary troubles that shape both child and parent. But Calvin loved his parents and appeared on track to live a successful and full life. This was before he became sick.

Because Jerri's love for her son was so deep and unwavering, she never doubted that when Calvin was first diagnosed with bipolar disorder, he would recover and everyone's life would return to what it had been. Jerri and her husband, Matt, would make certain of that outcome. With their help, Calvin would put this "blip" behind him. This is how their journey began, as it does for so many parents who love children with severe mental illness: with confidence, determination, and hope. Jerri sought good doctors and therapists to help quiet the storm in Calvin's brain. She learned everything she could about mania, depression, self-medication, and addiction that often accompany a bipolar diagnosis. Together with Matt, she believed they would help Calvin return to being the loving son they had raised.

But mental illness is cruel, persistent, and—when untreated—progressive.

Those of us who have a child with severe mental illness or addiction know what it is like to look into their face and see a stranger. It can feel as though an alien force has taken control. This loss is especially devastating when an adult child cannot accept the illness—an all-too-common symptom of the disease itself. There are moments of clarity. We hear our children promise that "this time" will be different. This time therapy will work. This time medication will help pull them back from the abyss. And slowly, painfully, we learn a truth no parent wants to face: recovery does not come in a straight line, it is never guaranteed, and it is not something a parent can control.

With each hospitalization and each arrest—and there were many of both—recovery seemed more distant. It was as if Jerri were trying to catch smoke with her fingers. The good times grew fewer; the bad times more frequent. Calvin would beg for help and then push his parents away with cruel words. He told Jerri he loved her. He told her he hated her. As his illness progressed, Calvin cut his parents out of his life and became homeless. How does a mother sleep at night knowing her son is wandering the streets?

What Jerri was experiencing, though she did not yet have the language for it, is what family therapist Pauline Boss calls *ambiguous loss*. Calvin was physically present but increasingly psychologically absent—a form of loss common in families affected by mental illness, addiction, dementia, and traumatic brain injury. There was no clear line between presence and absence, no socially recognized ending, and therefore no roadmap for grieving. Jerri was expected to hope and mourn at the same time—to hold on and let go simultaneously.

While many Americans with bipolar disorder receive treatment and are able to move forward with their lives, not everyone does. Calvin died at age twenty-three, despite the herculean efforts of his parents. He left behind unanswered questions, lingering doubts, and—most painfully for Jerri—no closure. The rituals that usually help people mourn proved ineffective. As Pauline Boss explains, ambiguous loss defies the ceremonies, language, and social acknowledgment that help make loss bearable.

Jerri came to realize that ambiguous loss had entered her life long before Calvin died. Throughout his four years struggling with severe mental illness, he was often physically present but psychologically absent. Like dementia or traumatic brain injury, mental illness had taken her son from her in pieces.

I had never heard the term *ambiguous loss* before I met Jerri. But when I read this book—with its skilled, compassionate writing and its clear-eyed exploration of unresolved grief—I thought about the death of my sister, Alice. She was killed in an automobile accident at seventeen while riding a motorbike I owned, on her way to visit a high school friend. A car struck her as both entered a blind rural intersection bordered by tall crops. I was two years younger and knew nothing about grief.

At her funeral, the minister quoted the Apostle Paul: "O death, where is your victory? O death, where is your sting?" That verse—and the well-meaning platitudes offered by friends ("This is part of God's plan." "She's in a better place." "Everything happens for a reason.")—rang hollow. At home, I watched my parents suffer. Even near the end of their lives—both lived to be ninety-four—you could not mention my sister's name without reopening their pain.

Pauline Boss describes a second form of ambiguous loss—one in which a loved one is physically absent but psychologically present. Although my sister died suddenly, her absence never resolved into anything resembling closure. Decades later, she remains vividly alive in my mind, in my parents' unhealed grief, and in my own longing. Her death, too, remained ambiguous.

Nineteen years after Alice's death, I woke one night calling out her name. The feelings I had buried as a child—silenced because her death was too painful for my parents to discuss—came spilling out. Seeking closure, I returned to the rural intersection where she was killed, hoping to make sense of my loss. Instead, I found only frustration, anger, and bewilderment. The sadness my parents carried daily had been passed on to me, settling in as an unwanted guest, forever present.

That is why I am so grateful to Jerri Clark for writing *Gone Before Gone*. After Calvin's death, she did not fall silent. She became an advocate for others living with severe mental illness. That is how we first met—as parents demanding that our nation build a more humane and effective mental health care system. Her tireless efforts locally, statewide, and nationally through Treatment Advocacy Center—an organization dedicated to removing barriers to treatment—created an immediate bond between us.

Jerri's determination and search for meaning led her to Pauline Boss and the teaching that ambiguous loss does not require resolution. With the same passion she brings to advocacy, Jerri found solace in understanding loss and became determined to share that understanding with others. Reading this book helped me realize that the grief I carry—for my sister's death, my son's mental illness, my father's dementia—does not need to be fixed. Instead, it needs to be acknowledged, named, and lived with.

As Boss teaches, the goal is not closure but resilience: learning to live fully while holding unanswered questions, fractured narratives, and enduring love.

Gone Before Gone is a gift because it offers permission to stop asking the impossible of ourselves. By sharing Calvin's life, his death, and her own journey through grief, Jerri Clark shows us that while we may never move on from loss, we can live well alongside it. Perhaps that, ultimately, is both Calvin's legacy—and hers.

—Pete Earley, author of *Crazy: A Father's Search*
Through America's Mental Health Madness,
finalist for the 2007 Pulitzer Prize

Preface
By Calvin Clark

Postmarked January 16, 2018, from Seattle, Washington.

Dear Mom,

I'm writing you after our good encounter today, Sunday, as you head off on your work trip. Hoping this letter gets to you as you get home.

Ever since I withdrew from classes at Willamette and was diagnosed with bipolar disorder, nothing has been the same. I know now that my diagnosis and subsequent mentally ill behavior caused great discord in our family. That is my responsibility. I was 19 years old when trouble started brewing, an adult in our world. Because of decisions that I made and behaviors that I exhibited, I caused you and Dad great pain. I am truly and deeply sorry.

Since things started going South, I have experienced mental institution no fewer than ten times, jail three times, and homelessness three times. By all accounts, I should be dead, or down and out, or otherwise disabled. But you and Dad have bailed me out, fixed me up, and stayed on my team through everything. For all of your patience, love, kindness, and generosity, thank you!!!

There are things I've said that I wish I could take back. I know I've said I hate you. I know I've said you're the worst person. I know I've made you my enemy. I don't mean any of it. I don't think any of that. I love you, you're the best person, and you are my ally.

I'm so happy for you and excited for you with all of the great new work you've been doing. I'm so proud to call you my mom. I'm also just plain old regular proud!

You and Dad gave me an excellent childhood. We took vacations, went to the beach, played games, watched movies (all the right genres and all the right movies), went to grandparents' houses, surfed, skied . . . I could go on. I was never hungry. I was never cold. I had great teachers at top schools and made good friends. When I think of my childhood I think of a smiling sun in a cutely drawn neighborhood—everything a kid could ever want. I often brag that every house in our neighborhood had exactly two trees in front of it.

As I grew up . . . I had lots of fun, great friendships, newfound freedom. I deeply cherished my later years of high school, with huge debate wins and straight A's all the way up until that last semester; perhaps that's when I first became depressed . . . and [during college] it's as if my very mind was ripped open, even pulled apart at the seam (I guess that would be the corpus colosseum).

Now, I fit the standard diagnostics for a mental patient who is bipolar. There are some things I want to clarify. I "carry the diagnosis of bipolar disorder." I myself am not bipolar. What I mean is that I am so much more than some mental illness created by doctors. I am a Divine Being, an intellectual, a speaker, a writer, a healer, a leader, a teacher, and a friend. I am a son, a grandson, a brother, and a brother-in-law. There are so many great "I am" statements the last thing anybody needs to be thinking about me is, "Oh, he's bipolar."

No! With medication, therapy, stable housing, employment, income, friends, family, my poetry book, my spirituality, and everything else that I have going for me, I am mentally well. I am mentally well. There's also a lot more healing that I need. Relationships to build, relationships to mend. I'm working on that too.

I'm just so excited for the future. I have big business ventures brewing—advertising, tutoring, healing. . . .

I'm in a place now where I'm ready to build community, new friendships, a house for myself. I'm going to stop losing things, cherish gifts more, keepsakes and family heirlooms. I have a picture of all four of us when Michelle and I were young. That is precious to me. I've even thought about going back to school and finishing this time! I want to major in English.

I'm very hopeful and even (ironically) cheery regarding "I Hope I Die on a Monday and Other Morbidly Optimistic Poems," my upcoming poetry book. I want to have it published in paper, illustrated and all. This will be a crowning achievement of my life, to be a published author.

Mom, you and Dad are really just the best. I wish there was a word to say, "I love you. I'm sorry, and thank you" all at once. You will always be my mom, and I will always be your son. May we know peace and joy, great love and bliss in all our many years to come. I am so happy to be alive. It is such a blessing to just exist. I love you so much.

Always, Calvin

Ambiguity

Life's only clarity was sheer uncertainty.
I had nothing to hold, and so I fell. Nothing
would ever help me thrive, survive. Just confusion.

My hopes were abandoned, a useless tool to me.
And my grief was homeless, like my still-so-young son.
There was no hospice house for comforting our kind.

Furious at a world that stood by while he died,
By degrees. First his mind, then his body followed.
My losses were a weight, awaiting nothingness.

From a bottomless well, I knew that unknowing
Was my only way up and out of this darkness.
Curiosity then, a choice to look around.

I could no longer cling to the life I had planned.
A timid voice hinted, "Here . . . use this map instead."
There were lots of arrows, pointed every which way.

The choice was just to choose, go somewhere, do something.
Somehow share my truth and tell someone what's happened.
Just an echo at first, my own screams through a void.

But then there was a shift, and I wasn't alone.
Other weary travelers have baggage just like mine.
Loved ones lost in their minds, beings gone before gone.

Taken by illnesses, then abandoned to fail.
How to reconcile this, a living death, not death?
I tasted that grief first, before this bitter kind.

Like families hurt by war, we count our battle scars.
All our losses are real. They have meaning and heft.
By naming them we can begin to journey on.

I rediscovered sky by gazing at wet sand.
I rediscovered sound by listening to silence.
My new life became full because I've been emptied.

Life's only clarity is sheer uncertainty.
We have nothing to hold, and so we fall. We all
Help each other thrive, survive this confusion.

—*Jerri Niebaum Clark*
Written in honor of Calvin Clark's thirtieth birthday, November 28, 2025

CONTENTS

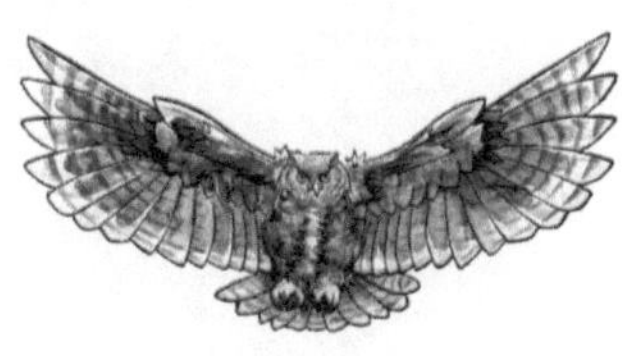

Part 1

Orientation